Essentials of Pilates

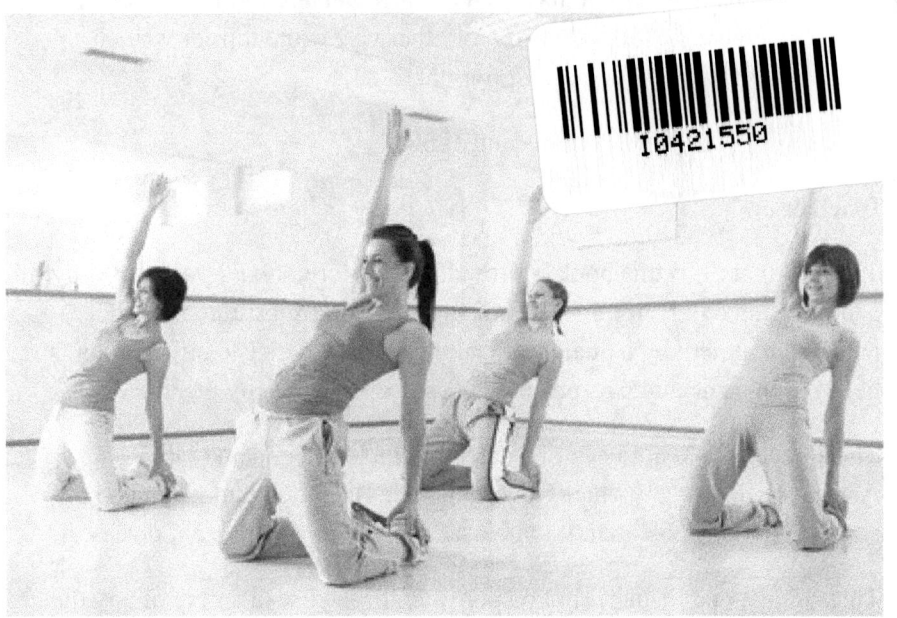

Health Learning Series

M. Usman

Mendon Cottage Books

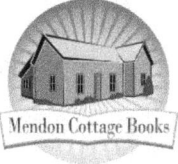

JD-Biz Publishing

All Rights Reserved.

Disclaimer

The information is this book is provided for informational purposes only. It is not intended to be used and medical advice or a substitute for proper medical treatment by a qualified health care provider. The information is believed to be accurate as presented based on research by the author.

The contents have not been evaluated by the U.S. Food and Drug Administration or any other Government or Health Organization and the contents in this book are not to be used to treat cure or prevent disease.

The author or publisher is not responsible for the use or safety of any diet, procedure, or treatment mentioned in this book. The author or publisher is not responsible for errors or omissions that may exist.

Warning

The Book is for informational purposes only and before taking on any diet, treatment, or medical procedure, it is recommended to consult with your primary health care provider.

Our books are available at

1. Amazon.com
2. Barnes and Noble
3. Itunes
4. Kobo
5. Smashwords
6. Google Play Books

Table of Contents

Getting Started

Chapter #1 – What is Pilates?

I'm sure getting your hands dirty with the various techniques of Pilates would be the first thing on your mind, but, before we go into that, you should know the main focus of Pilates, its origin, and the idea behind Pilates.

Pilates was developed in the mid-20th century by German-born fitness enthusiast, Joseph Pilates. He developed this system when he was in England during World War 1, originally to rehabilitate the injured war prisoners. So, the roots of today's modern Pilates lie in the camps of England. He started it all with the idea that he should fix mattress springs to the wall, the design of these springs would mimic the body muscles, and it would help people heal. Joseph Pilates named his fitness program "Contrology". Pilates continued to make innovative and appropriate improvements in his methodology, until his death. After realizing the fact that these exercises can increase mental well-being and fitness levels of a normal individual, Pilates entered the mainstream around the world as an efficient and practicable work out type. Right after its development, Pilates was not very famous among the people, and it didn't get the due importance until 21st century. Pilates gained popularity in the early years of the 21st century, especially in United States. Now many people from all over the world are practicing Pilates, either individually or at a Pilates Centre.

What kinds of exercises does it involve?

The answer to this question is that Pilates is basically an exercise methodology that is adapted for the sake of muscular strength, endurance movements, and low-impact flexibility. Expanding the discussion further, Pilates comprises of a series of controlled and definite movements, involving more than 500 controlled workouts. It makes groups of several muscles work at the same time with the help of continuous and even motions. The particular concentration lies in stabilizing and strengthening the core muscles. It mainly emphasizes the use of thighs, hips, lower back, and abdominals for core strength. In Pilates, the main focus lies on the quality of motion instead of its quantity. This means performing steps at a slower pace and less repetitions with control and precise movements are more important than the number of steps. If an individual wants to extract maximum benefits from Pilates, performance of each and every movement accurately is necessary. This is the main reason that many of the individuals find Pilates to be so useful. Most people want to enhance their sport or activity level, so they turn to Pilates, because it uses a balanced approach. It does not make a specific muscle group overwork, and the body is capable to work as a holistic and efficient system in sports, as well as in daily life activities. It also encourages strength of bones and joints by utilizing body weight as a resistance.

To an individual, Pilates may sound terrifying, but if you want to build strength in your core muscles for balance and flexibility in your body, Pilates is one of the best accessible ways. It also helps you to improve your body posture. Many individuals want an exercise type that will complement their weight training exercises and/or aerobic exercises, and Pilates provides an excellent option.

What age group of people should follow Pilates? Is it for injured people? Is it for people who are suffering from debilitating diseases? The answer is that Pilates is a type of exercise that is designed for people over the entire age spectrum to promote fitness level among individuals. Moreover, it is equally beneficial and efficient for people who have suffered from any injuries or who are suffering from diseases such as low back pain, osteoporosis, and arthritis.

Chapter #2 – Concept behind Pilates

After discussing the brief history of Pilates, you must be eager to know the various concepts associated with Pilates. Many of you may be concerned about Pilates involving some kind of religious concepts like Yoga. Unlike yoga, Pilates is an exercise that totally lacks the religious and spiritual concepts. Until now, many of you may be thinking that Yoga and Pilates is the same thing, but this isn't so. Yoga and Pilates are two different streams of exercises. Coming back to our topic of concern, we have six major principles associated with Pilates. Keeping the fact in mind that Joseph Pilates did not directly propose the Pilates principles, you should know that today's Pilates concepts have been derived from Joseph Pilates' work by the set of instructions proposed by later instructors. This is the root cause of disagreement about the order of principles, number of principles, and the particular terms associated with different concepts of Pilates. However, the set of six principles that I am going to present you here can be found in many versions of Pilates principles. I can assure you that these six fundamental principles are the basics that you should be aware of if you want to be a part of any Pilates program.

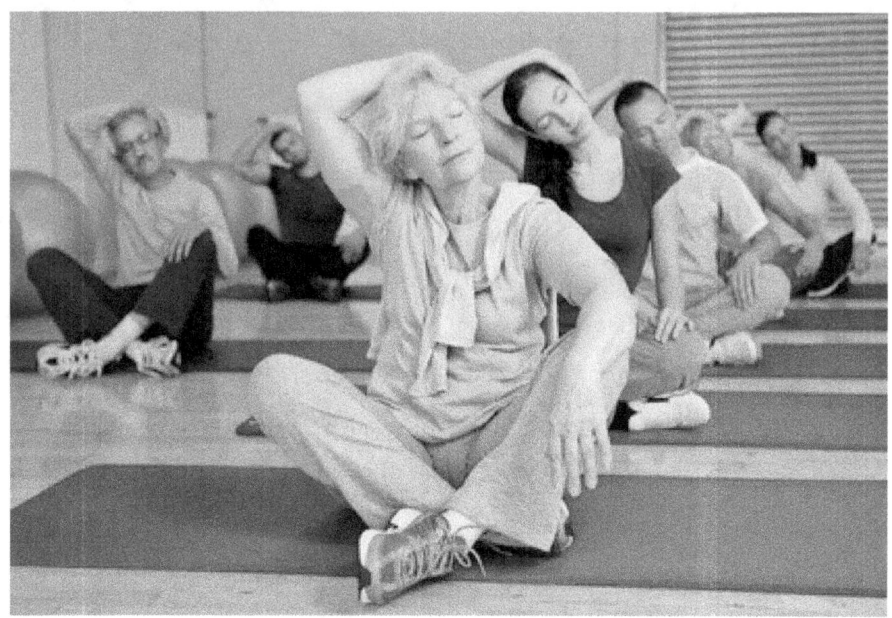

Major principles of Pilates:

- **Center focus:**

This concept demands that the body to pay attention to body centering, or, in other words, concentrating on centering the core. The particular term that is used for this body center in Pilates is powerhouse area. In these centering exercises, the specific area of the body that is in use lies in the space present between the lower ribs and the pubic bone. So, the main design of Pilates exercise is to make a workout from the center of your body that is powerhouse to the rest of body.

- **Concentration:**

If you want to extract the maximum benefit out of Pilates, then your body should be able to concentrate. The concept "concentration" in Pilates concepts is the one having the most importance in this work out type. So, I must say, that in order to achieve best results, you must pay due concentration to each and every motion of yours that you are performing during each exercise. Though concentration is the main concept behind getting the maximum benefit, you must show your commitment by involving yourself in a regular scheduled program.

- **Ability to control:**

Is only concentration enough for a Pilates workout? The answer is no, only concentration doesn't work for Pilates. After you have successfully concentrated on your motions, you should be able to control them as well. Exercises that are done without proper control of the body parts are thought to produce the minimum benefit. However, control over your body parts that are involved in workouts, and control over the body parts that do not appear to be directly involved in exercises, are both equally important. After all, mental control seems to be very difficult to obtain without any physical control over the movements. So, it is advised to practice control over the entire body.

- **Precise motions:**

Now that you are able to concentrate and control your motions, you must be capable of developing a system consisting of precise movements that are designed to leave a maximum effect on your body muscles. The motions must not be performed to the maximum efficiency, nor should they be performed to such a small degree that they do not leave any positive impact on the body. While you are doing a workout, three basic terms should always be on your mind:

- Proper placement

- Alignment of one body part relative to another

- Trajectory for each body part

- **Breath control:**

Breath control and regularity both have utmost importance in every mental piece of exercise. Joseph Pilates laid special emphasis on using a very full and deep breath in his workouts. The breathing process in Pilates is similar to any other slow exercise program. You must exhale when you are pushing weight, and while releasing weight you must inhale. Consider an example here: while you are doing bicep curls, you would take a deep breath first, and then you would exhale while pulling the dumbbell towards your body. The same technique works for Pilates. In fact, Pilates workouts are coordinated with breathing techniques. So, we can regard proper breathing a fundamental part of Pilates.

- **Flow:**

The sixth fundamental principle associated with Pilates is the flow at which workouts are carried out. Like all other exercises, the three main goals applied by Pilates are:

- Fluidity

- Graceful approach

- Ease

Now many of you would be thinking that "control" and "flow" are overlapping to some extent. Well, you are thinking right, because this concept of "flow" is very closely related to control, in which all controlled movements are through grace and fluidity. The energy gained while doing exercises connects all the body parts, and then the energy is circulated in an even way throughout the body. It is said that if one loses flow and control, Pilates equipment is just machines giving you no proper benefit.

Chapter #3 – Equipment Required for Pilates

By this point, many of our readers might be thinking that Pilates is quite a difficult task to do, especially exercising with fluidity and control. So, here we have the best way to practice Pilates by using Pilates Equipment. The purpose of designing this equipment is to mimic the proper motions, in order to meet the Pilates concepts presented in the last section of book.

The types of Pilates machines available in market vary from the level of beginners to expert. You should select the equipment according to your experience. In the beginning, you do not need any mechanical device. Your chair, ring, and table will work for your simple exercises. Anyhow, if you want to select machines for complicated exercises, you must seek professional help. In the market, there are many items available that will trick you into thinking that you must have this equipment for your Pilates workouts. In general, all equipment is meant for the support of the body, while focusing on making your exercises more effective. Any item that is promising you to melt the pounds away faster than the normal process is not a good choice. The success in Pilates solely depends on the control over your body and the performance of the movements fluidly and smoothness. So, I suggest that you invest your money only in the equipment that will protect your body from injuries and equipment that serves as a supporting device.

If you want your Pilates program to be successful, you should know about the following equipment that is often required:

- **Pilates Machines:**

This device is available for advanced Pilates exercise. There are certain complicated motions that you cannot perform with the body alone, so you must need a machine for such complicated motions. When you are using a Pilates machine, you can think of it as a mechanical device provided with a pulley system and a variety of cloth straps. Anyhow, the fact about a Pilates machine is that this machine is hardly ever used in the balanced programs.

- **Pilates Table:**

This is a specially designed table with the purpose of supporting the body when it performs movements involving elevation of some of the body parts. Any well-built table can be used for the same purpose. You must make sure that the table is in good condition and is strong enough to prevent any breaks or falls that can cause injuries. In addition, the table chosen should be able to provide enough support and cushioning to keep your joints and bones relaxed.

- **Pilates Chair:**

This is a specially designed supporting device meant to lift up the buttocks above the legs, as the individual sits in any manner. Generally, these stools are designed on an incline so that they make the sitting position more comfortable. The chair selected by you should be high enough to provide suitable cushioning and proper elevation, to make the movements easy.

- **Pilates Rings:**

This device was invented by Joseph Pilates, the original founder of Pilates, with a purpose of increasing the resistance to some of the movements. These rings can result in an increase in the potential for workouts to develop muscles, rather than just focusing on flexibility. If you want to use Pilates for more than a single reason, I suggest you to invest your money in Pilates Rings.

- **Exercise Ball:**

Only a few exercises of Pilates require these devices. If you have an exercise ball, you are already set for performing those exercises that need it in Pilates. On the other hand, if you do not have an exercise ball, you shouldn't worry about it. Your instructor will tell you when you will need the exercise ball.

- **Pilates Mats:**

Pilates mats are quite inexpensive and they are meant to support and cushion the body. Their core purpose is to avoid discomfort when you are practicing Pilates on hard surfaces. You can easily get Pilates mats from retail stores dealing with exercise or sporting goods. Mats are necessary for most of the Pilates exercises.

- **Pilates Bolster:**

This is a cheap supporting mechanism that is usually meant to support the spine when complicated movements are performed. Pilates bolsters help to make movements more relaxing and comfortable rather than preventing injury.

- **Clothing:**

As far as the clothing is concerned, it is advised to wear comfortable clothes that are not too tight or loose. The issue with the tight clothes is that they can be uncomfortable and can also cause embarrassing rips. With the loose clothing, the problem is that they can cause trips and can get caught in machines. However, some of the Pilates practitioners recommend to wear tight clothes for maximum mobility during workouts, but these are a supplement rather than a requirement.

- **Music:**

Ambient sounds are of vital importance for some people when they are practicing Pilates. This is acceptable only when the music does not distract your concentration from the workouts. Instead of heavy metal or rock music, using a compact disc of a small stream or rainfall is recommended. There are many pre-recorded sessions available for you. One additional benefit of purchasing the Pilates music is that they usually have recordings of time sections that will let you know that it's time to move towards the next exercise.

Benefits of Pilates

Pilates is an excellent exercise type for everyone. It provides you both physical and mental benefits of good health. That's why experts recommend incorporating Pilates or Yoga as part of your daily routine. Pilates is the type of exercise that you can adapt on daily basis, knowing that your joints, skeletal structure, or soft tissue won't get over stressed. Some of the physical and mental benefits achieved through Pilates are listed below:

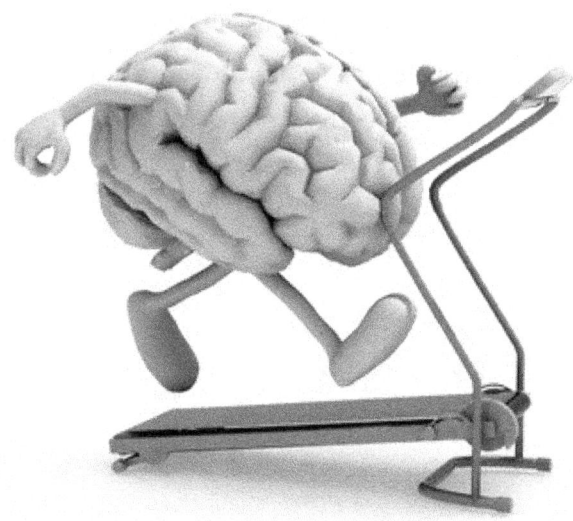

Physical Benefits:

- **Lowers Blood Pressure:**

Studies have revealed that if you have high blood pressure problems, Pilates workout will bring it back to a normal level.

- **Stretching:**

If you are suffering from any injury, Pilates will assist you in the recovery from this injury. In fact, participants have reported that several injuries can be healed in a comparatively lesser amount of time. A survey was conducted to explore the injuries type where Pilates was proved to be beneficial in reducing the heeling time. The results are as follows:

- 50% had back injuries

- 35% had knee injuries

- 7% had arms injuries

- 5% had shoulder injuries

- 3% had neck injuries

- **Minimizes pain associated with Arthritis:**

Pilates has proved to be very beneficial in reducing the pain associated with arthritis.

- **Strengthens the Immune System:**

Studies have revealed that regular Pilates practitioners have much stronger immune systems as compared to those who do not practice Pilates exercises.

- **Reduced Muscle Tension:**

People suffering from tense muscles or joints have reported Pilates to be quite a valuable agent in the reduction of these tensed body parts.

- **Reduction in Headaches:**

Pilates has been reported to reduce headaches and sometimes migraines as well. Regularly following Pilates may remove the pain or at least give you a long break from it.

- **Facilitates Weight Loss:**

Pilates is particularly very helpful for people who want to lose weight. Studies have shown that Pilates is very effective in controlling the ideal weight levels.

- **Increased Lung Function and Capacity:**

Pilates can improve airflow and increase the lung capacity due to the deep and smooth breathing steps associated with Pilates. According to a wind musician's survey, Pilates can improve lung capacity up to 5% in only two weeks of regular practice.

- **Lowers Cholesterol Level:**

According to a recent survey, people following Pilates on a regular basis have much lower cholesterol levels. This is due to the apparent mental control associated with Pilates.

- **Improved Central Nervous System Functionality:**

Pilates can afford lower amounts of electrical activity in the brain resulting in the increased function of the central nervous system. It also makes the reaction time faster.

- **Improved Breathing Regularity:**

Your breathing becomes more regular, as you control your breathing while doing a Pilates workout. As a result, any kind of activity can become 56% more effective.

- **Reduction in Symptoms Associated with Illness:**

According to a study, people having chronic diseases such as asthma, obesity, or AIDS found out that exercising Pilates in a weight loss regime really relieved these diseases symptoms.

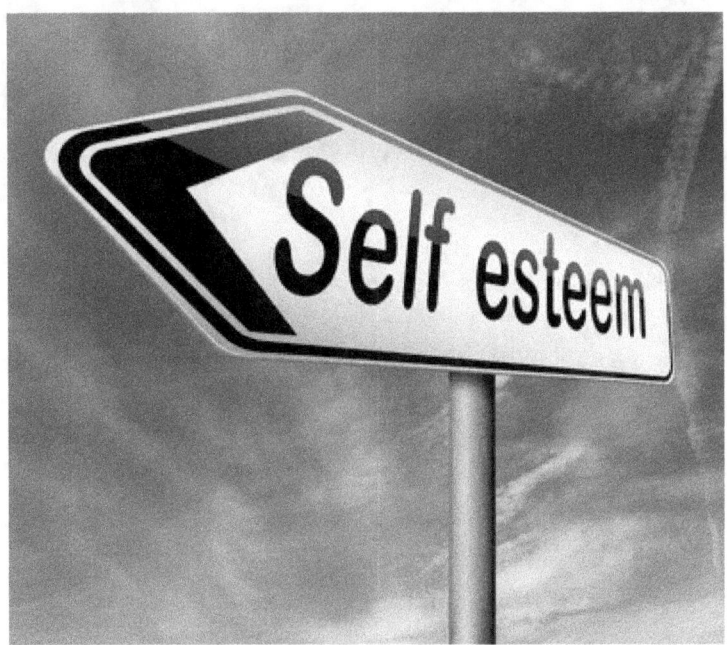

Mental Benefits:

Some of the mental benefits associated with Pilates are listed below:

- Reduction of Anxiety

- Motivation

- Increased focus and concentration

- Emotional Stability

- Improvement of Memory

- Improved Problem Solving Abilities

- Improved Intelligence Capability

- Reduction in Insomnia

- Improved Sleep Patterns

- Promotes Mental Stability, Will Power, and the Elimination of bad Habits

- Increase in the Release of Serotonin

- Improved Stability in Relationships

Pilates Exercises

Chapter #1 – The Fundamentals

In the present world, you will observe fantastic changes in the way Pilates exercises are performed. A traditional order is observed in Pilates exercises, developed by Joseph Pilates himself. Ten moves of classical Pilates mat exercises are listed below:

- **Begin with Pilates Fundamentals:**

In the beginning, you need to warm yourself up before starting this exercise. This is the fundamental rule to beginning Pilates. After warming yourself up, you can engage your body in a Pilates workout.

- **The Hundred:**

This move is used to build stamina, core strength, and coordination. For performing this work out, you must fully engage your abdominal muscles, while you practice a dynamic breathing pattern. You may make modifications for the sake of your ease. These modifications include working with the legs higher and leaving the head down.

- **The Roll Up:**

This move is a great challenge for your abdominal muscles and a fantastic support for spine. It is said that one well-performed Roll Up is equal, in its effect, to six regular sit-ups. If you want a flat stomach, the Roll Up is much better than crunches.

- **The Roll Over:**

Joseph Pilates saw this exercise as stimulating the spine. It involves a lot of spinal articulation and the only way to control it is that you should control your abdominal muscles. Keep it in mind that the Roll Over can go only as far as the shoulders. It does not involve the rolling up of your neck.

- **One Leg Circle:**

One leg circle aims for core stability. One must keep the entire trunk, including the hips portion steady as one leg circles independently. In case you need some modifications, keep the non-working leg bent with the foot flat on the floor. You can also slightly bend the knee of your working leg.

- **Rolling like a Ball:**

It is the first of the rolling exercises. This move stimulates your spine and deeply works for your abdominals. Rolling like a ball tunes your inner flow of movement and breath in your body. Modifications can be made by holding your thighs behind the knees and opening your legs further out from the body. However, if you have neck or back problems, do not do rolling exercises.

- **Single Leg Stretch:**

This move is considered a workout that targets your lower abs. this exercise works the entire core and it requires strength and stamina, as you have to maintain your upper body in a curve and keep the trunk stable while you switch the arm and leg positions. You can modify this exercise by keeping your head down and working with your legs higher.

- **Double Leg Stretch:**

For attaining more abdominal endurance and strength, single leg stretch is followed by double leg stretch. Double leg stretch is the way through which you can experience working from the center of body, while your legs and arms reach away and return together.

- **Spine Stretch:**

It is a Pilates mat exercise that will feel really good. It is a flexion exercise that is done with the abs lifted. It mainly emphasizes stretching the spine. Spine stretch may also result in the stretching of your hamstrings. It also provides a moment to center yourself before you move to the next challenging exercise. Spine stretch does not need modifications often, but people having tight hamstrings may sit on a small lift and may bend their knees slightly. You may also do Spine stretch with your arms lower and fingertips along the floor.

- **Open Leg Rocker:**

This exercise is meant for deep abdominal control. The required rolling will come from deep within the core. It can't be achieved from momentum. You must not throw your head back to get going, nor should you jerk yourself up by pulling on the legs. Rolling exercises can be very hard for some and some people can't perform rolling exercises because of their back pains. Anyhow, you can find open leg balance in an alternative to open leg rocker.

Chapter #2 – Exercise Modification Tips

Modification is regarded as one of the essential elements of a Pilates workout. You can make your exercise less or more difficult through appropriate modifications. Modifications can also be adjusted to compensate for physical limitations, if you have any. If you have any particular physical issue, you must inform your instructor about it before class. A good instructor will offer you modifications and will be able to tailor an appropriate modification for you.

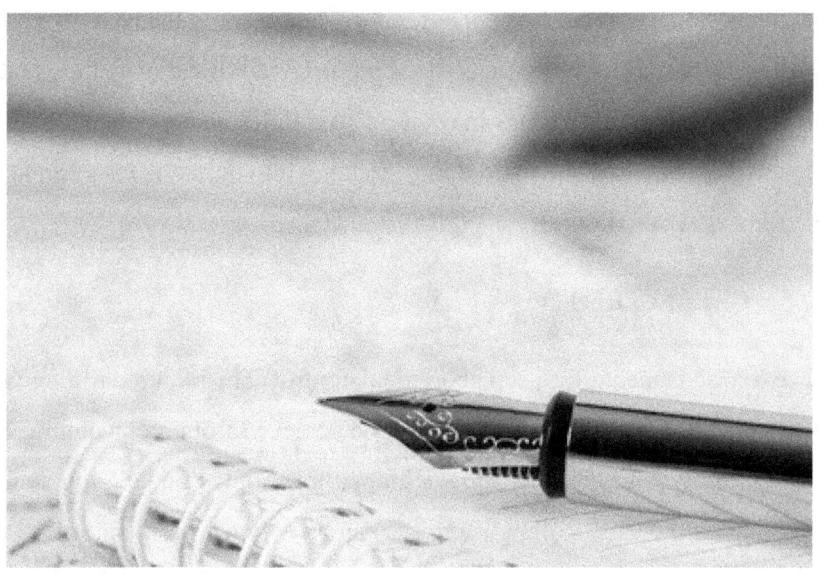

- **A good Warm Up is essential:**

It is very important to center yourself and warm up well before you launch yourself into more exhausting exercise. Pilates is a body-mind integrative practice as well as a physical training method. You should take your time to warm-up your body and mind up. This will make your Pilates workout even more effective for you.

- **Pay attention to the placement of your head:**

Your head is a heavy portion of your body. If you are suffering from back or neck problems, you have to leave your head down when exercising on your back or front. You will be able to support your head and neck with much less strain once you have developed a lot of core strength. Sample exercises that are found effective with the head down include:

- Single Leg Stretch

- The Hundred

You should treat your head and neck as extensions of your spine. If you are using your belly, you should lift your head as the extension of the spine and do not break at your neck. When you curve forward during a flexion exercise, take care not to over tuck your chin and continue your spine curve with your neck.

- **Protect your neck and upper spine:**

You can do some of the exercises in a much better way by using a neck roll or a low pillow for the support of your head. You may want to put the cushion up on the reformer. However, if you are lifting your head up or rolling back, you must not have a pad under your neck or the reformer head rest up. For instance, if you are doing a roll over, you will not have a pillow under your neck. Rolling exercises, such as rolling like a ball and open leg rocker, are considered to be standard moves in Pilates mat exercises. However, if you are suffering from back or neck problems, you should skip the rolling portion of these exercises and should use them as balancing challenges as an alternative.

- **Your Arms are heavy:**

Your arms are heavy just like your head. The exercise becomes more challenging as you stretch your arms away from the body. For example, in a roll down, it will not stress the neck and back to cross your arms across your chest rather than leaving them outstretched. If you want to make your exercise more difficult for completing the challenge you are after, using the arms as leverage is a good technique. For example, you can do many exercises in the sidekick series by keeping your top arm away from the mat. In fact, you can make appropriate safety choices for your body even in the class.

- **Bend your knees to protect your back:**

Pilates exercises that are done on the back have a common progression of keeping the knees bent and feet flat on the floor. This gives a good position to work the upper body portion. Once you have built sufficient abdominal strength, your legs can move to table top position, where your knees are bent and shins are parallel to floor. To keep the pelvis and legs stable, there is a lower abs challenge. Finally, you can move to the full extension of legs. Following this progression, you can develop many Pilates exercises suitable for you. If you are fully aware of these positions, you can use the exercise that is right for you.

- **Low legs increase the challenge:**

You have to examine the height of your legs first. If you have outstretched your legs in the air, the lower they are, the harder your abdominals have to work. If you lower yourself and your back starts to arch, your legs are too low and you are putting strain on your back. It is always advisable to perform exercise by keeping the legs a little higher until you have developed sufficient abdominal strength to protect your back. Afterwards, you can start the workout with the legs held in a lower position.

- **If you have tight hamstrings:**

Many people have tight hamstrings that provide resistance in sitting up with ease with their legs straight out. If you have tight hamstrings, you can use one of the following methods to work out:

- Put a small lift under your hips

- Place a folded towel under your hips

- Foam wedge can also be used

- **Wrist pain in weight bearing exercises:**

Many people are confronted with wrist pains when doing weight bearing exercises. So, it is better for them to keep a folded Pilates rubber band or a foam wedge under the heel of the hand. This makes the weight bearing exercises easy by taking enough pressure off the wrist.

Chapter #3 –Workout with Pilates Ring, Ball & Band

For making your exercises more effective, you can use Pilates rings, an exercise ball, and resistance bands in your workouts. This is a full body sequence and it will engage your core and it will focus on your arm and leg toning as well. If you do not have the required equipment, you can use certain other alternatives.

Warm Up – Palm Press with Pilates Ring:

- Firstly, you need to warm up your core with continuous engagement of the pelvic floor, upper back, chest, and abdominal muscles with full breathing.

- Sit tall with the legs crossed.

- Place the Pilates ring in front of you, put both of your palms on it, and inhale.

- Now exhale and as you press down the Pilates ring, use this exhale to engage yourself to the pelvic floor and pull your abdominal muscles in.

Roll Up with Pilates Ring:

- Keep your legs straight while you lie on your back.

- Keep your hands on either side of the Pilates ring and elevate your arms vertical to your shoulders, so that the ring becomes parallel to ceiling.

- Now inhale deeply.

- Exhale, keeping your ribs down and as you keep the ring overhead, let your shoulder blades slide down your back.

- Inhale and bring your arms and the ring forward as you start curling your upper body off the mat.

Leg Bend and stretch with the Resistance Band:

- Lie down on your back while bringing your legs in towards the chest, and place the resistance band around your feet soles.

- Put your feet in a configuration where the heels of your feet are together and the toes are slightly apart. By doing so, you have put your feet in a Pilates V.

- Inhale and then exhale engaging your abdominal muscles.

Single Leg Circle Exercise with Resistance Band:

- Keep your legs extended and together while you lie on your back.

- Now, move your one leg in toward your chest and surround your foot with the resistance bands.

- Now extend this leg towards the ceiling.

- With your outstretched leg, start making small circles.

- Only your outstretched leg should move in the hip socket, so use your abdominal muscles for the stability in the rest of your body.

- Inhale.

Bicep Curl with Resistance Band:

- This move is meant for arm exercise and it works for your abdominal muscles as well.

- Sit up tall, while your feet are flexed and wrapped around by a resistance band.

- Roll yourself down with a deep measure of abdominal muscles, so that your upper body is curled off and the lower back is on the mat.

- Inhale and extend the arms.

- Exhale and bring the arms to the start position.

Bridge on the Ball:

- Lie down on your back and keep your legs on the exercise ball, in a neutral spine position. You can bend your knees slightly.

- Keep your feet flexed.

- Keep your arms along your sides and pressed into the mat.

- Inhale.

- Exhale, while sending energy to your heals so that you can lift your hips up, making your shoulders, hips, and heels in a single straight line.

- Hold yourself for 10 seconds and breathe.

- Inhale and use your abdominal muscles to control the roll down.

Conclusion

Pilates is one of the best workouts and quite easily adaptable on a daily basis. Pilates is for the entire age spectrum and for all genders. It also works equally for injured people. You can get both physical and mental aspects of a healthy life from Pilates. The book starts out with the history of Pilates and slowly, but surely, goes into its techniques. The instructions have been provided in an easy-to-understand manner and can be followed by anyone who is enthusiastic about the activity. I hope that by the end of the book you have liked the content provided in this book, and that you agree that Pilates is one of the best exercises to do. Also, I really do hope that the book helps you conquer any fears and misconceptions you have about Pilates.

Thank you and best of luck!

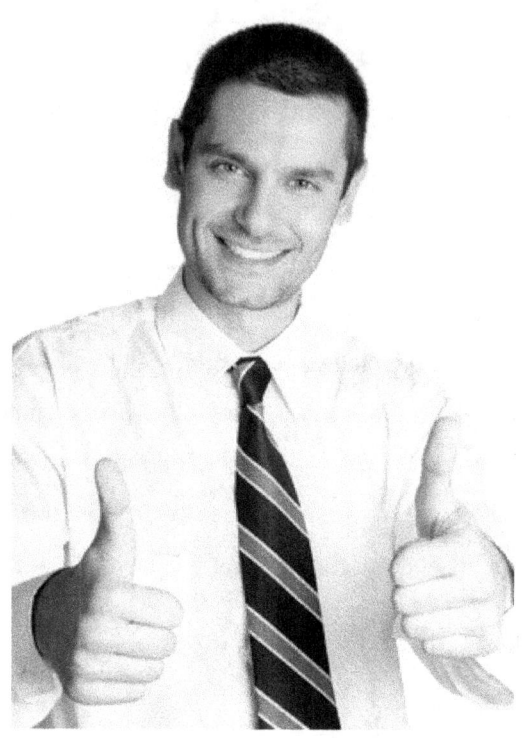

References

www.fotolia.com/id/51802921

www.fotolia.com/id/46908327

www.fotolia.com/id/45156048

www.fotolia.com/id/47169349

www.fotolia.com/id/52662791

www.fotolia.com/id/51102457

Author Bio

Muhammad Usman is a distinguished medical graduate of Allama Iqbal medical college (AIMC). He is a professional writer who has been in the field for more than 4 years. During this time he has produced 10,000+ articles, blogs, and eBooks on various niches related to diseases, health, fitness, nutrition, and well-being. He is a regular contributor to several journals related to medicine and surgery. He is the editor of several journals and newspapers.

Check out some of the other JD-Biz Publishing books

Gardening Series on Amazon

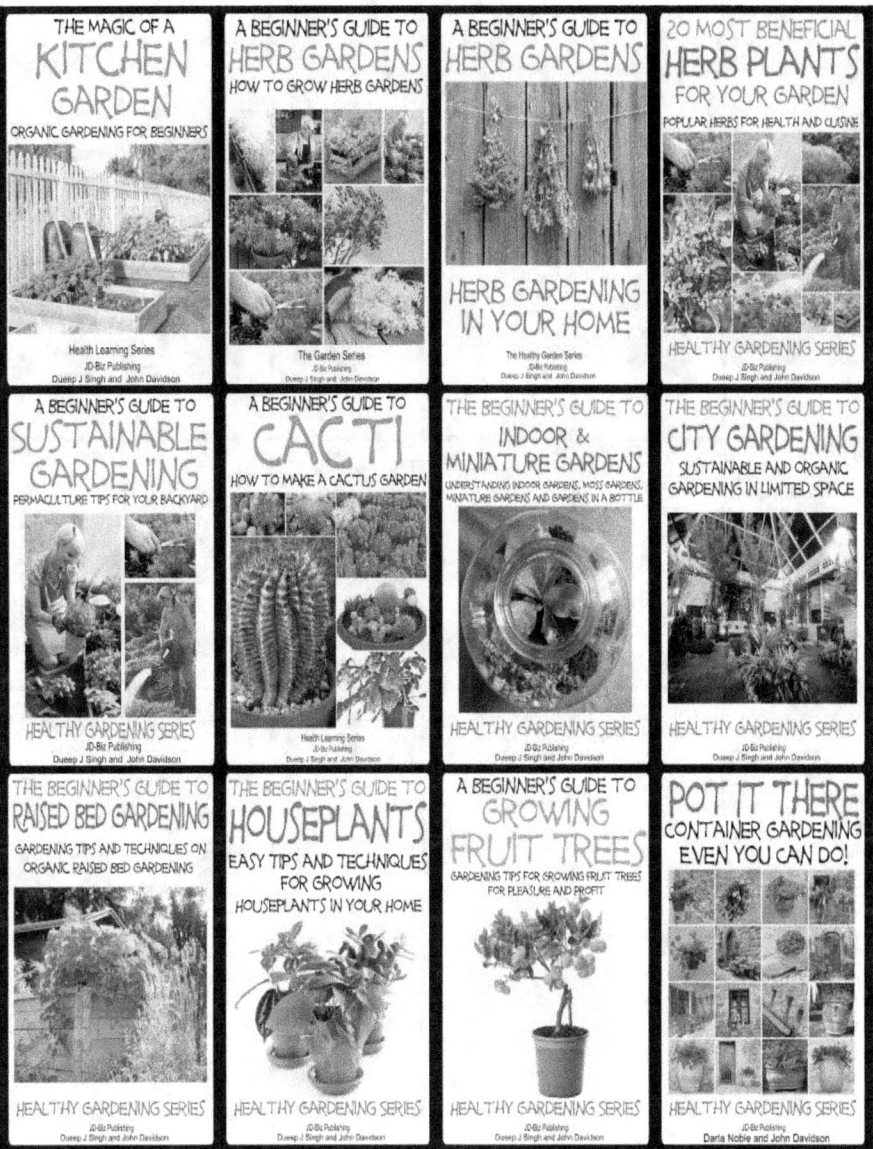

THE MAGIC OF GOOSEBERRIES FOR HEALTH AND BEAUTY
Natural Remedy Series
JD-Biz Publishing
Dueep J Singh and John Davidson

THE MAGIC OF YOGURT FOR COOKING AND BEAUTY
Natural Remedy Series
JD-Biz Publishing
Dueep J Singh and John Davidson

THE MAGIC OF LEMONS USING LEMONS FOR HEALTH AND BEAUTY
Natural Remedy Series
JD-Biz Publishing
Dueep J Singh and John Davidson

THE MAGIC OF CHILLIES FOR COOKING AND HEALING
Natural Remedy Series
JD-Biz Publishing
Dueep J Singh and John Davidson

THE MAGIC OF ONIONS ONIONS IN CUISINE TO CURE AND TO HEAL
Natural Remedy Series
JD-Biz Publishing
Dueep J Singh and John Davidson

THE MAGIC OF RADISHES TO CURE AND TO HEAL
Natural Remedy Series
JD-Biz Publishing
Dueep J Singh and John Davidson

THE MAGIC OF CARROTS TO CURE AND TO HEAL
Natural Remedy Series
JD-Biz Publishing
Dueep J Singh and John Davidson

THE HEALTH BENEFITS OF OREGANO FOR COOKING AND HEALTH
Natural Remedy Series
JD-Biz Publishing
M. Usman and John Davidson

THE MAGIC OF MARIGOLDS Marigolds for Health And Beauty
Natural Remedy Of
Natural Remedy Series
JD-Biz Publishing
Dueep J Singh and John Davidson

THE HEALTH BENEFITS OF CINNAMON
Natural Remedy Series
JD-Biz Publishing
M. Usman and J. Davidson

THE MAGIC OF COCONUTS FOR COOKING & HEALTH
Health Learning Series
JD-Biz Publishing
Dueep J Singh and John Davidson

THE MAGIC OF CLOVES FOR HEALING AND COOKING
Health Learning Series
JD-Biz Publishing
Dueep J Singh and John Davidson

THE MAGIC OF ASAFETIDA FOR COOKING AND HEALING
Health Learning Series
JD-Biz Publishing
Dueep J Singh and John Davidson

THE MAGIC OF NEEM MARGOSA TO HEAL
Natural Remedy Series
JD-Biz Publishing
Dueep J Singh and John Davidson

THE MAGIC OF SALT TO HEAL AND FOR BEAUTY
Natural Remedy Series
JD-Biz Publishing
Dueep J Singh and John Davidson

THE MAGIC OF POMEGRANATES FOR HEALTH AND BEAUTY
Natural Remedy Series
JD-Biz Publishing
Dueep J Singh and John Davidson

THE MAGIC OF DRY FRUIT AND SPICES REMEDIES AND RECIPES
Natural Remedy Series
JD-Biz Publishing
Dueep J Singh and John Davidson

THE HEALTH BENEFITS OF TURMERIC CURCUMIN FOR COOKING AND HEALTH
Natural Remedy Series
JD-Biz Publishing
M. Usman and J. Davidson

THE MAGIC OF ALOE VERA
Natural Remedy Series
JD-Biz Publishing
Dueep J Singh and John Davidson

THE MAGIC OF VEGETABLES ANCIENT HEALING REMEDIES AND TIPS
Natural Remedy Series
JD-Biz Publishing
Dueep J Singh and John Davidson

THE HEALTH BENEFITS OF ROSEMARY FOR COOKING AND HEALTH
Natural Remedy Series
JD-Biz Publishing
M. Usman and J. Davidson

THE MAGIC OF PEPPER & PEPPERCORNS FOR COOKING & HEALING
Natural Remedy Series
JD-Biz Publishing
Dueep J Singh and John Davidson

THE MAGIC OF MILK, BUTTER AND CHEESE FOR COOKING & HEALING
Natural Remedy Series
JD-Biz Publishing
Dueep J Singh and John Davidson

THE MAGIC OF CARDAMOMS FOR COOKING AND HEALTH
Health Learning Series
JD-Biz Publishing
Dueep J Singh and John Davidson

THE HEALTH BENEFITS OF BLACK CUMIN FOR COOKING AND HEALTH
Natural Remedy Series
JD-Biz Publishing
M. Usman and J. Davidson

THE MAGIC OF BASIL-TULSI TO HEAL NATURALLY
Health Learning Series
JD-Biz Publishing
Dueep J Singh and John Davidson

THE MAGIC OF SPICES FOR HEALTH AND CUISINE
Natural Remedy Series
JD-Biz Publishing
Dueep J Singh and John Davidson

THE MAGIC OF ROSES FOR COOKING AND BEAUTY
Natural Remedy Series
JD-Biz Publishing
Dueep J Singh and John Davidson

The Miraculous Healing Powers of GINGER
Natural Remedy Series
JD-Biz Publishing
Dueep J Singh and John Davidson

The Miracle of HONEY
Natural Remedy Series
JD-Biz Publishing
Dueep J Singh and John Davidson

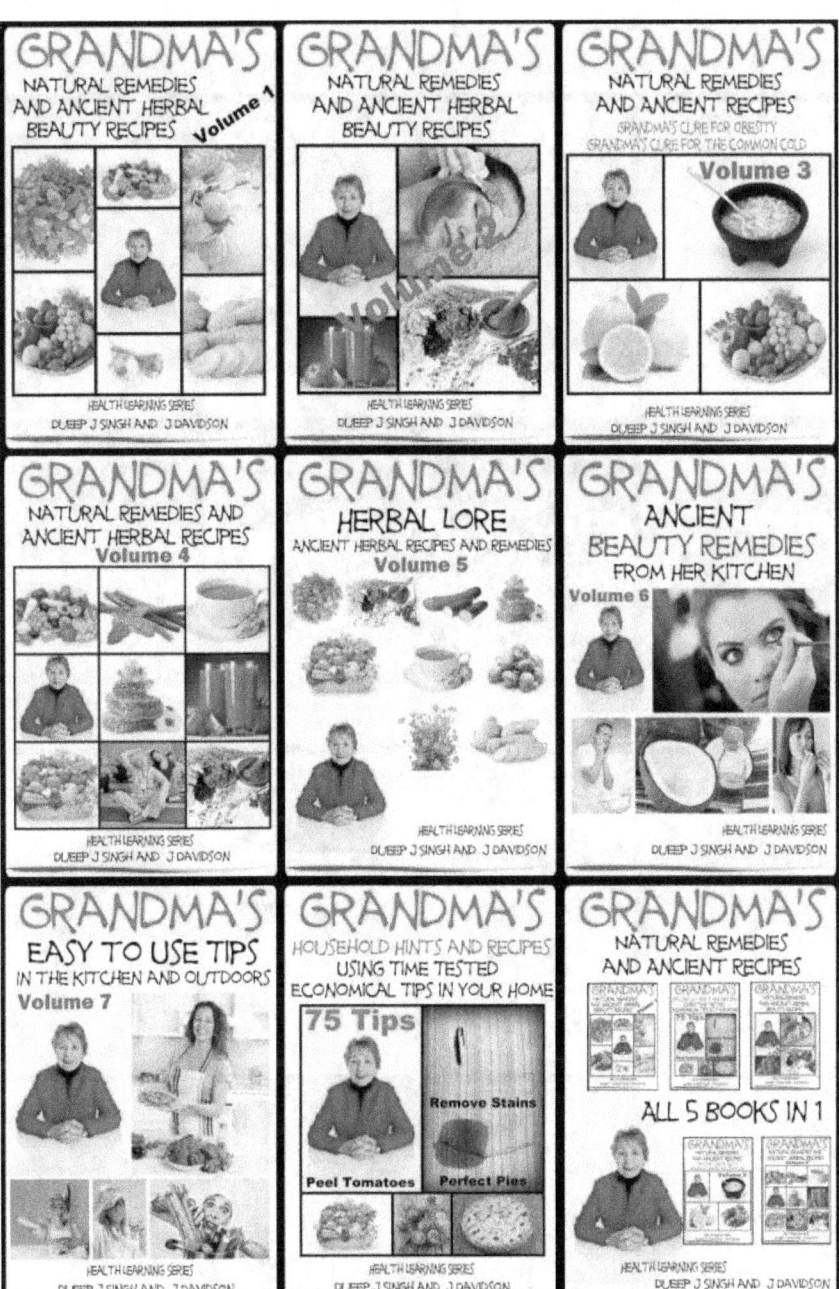

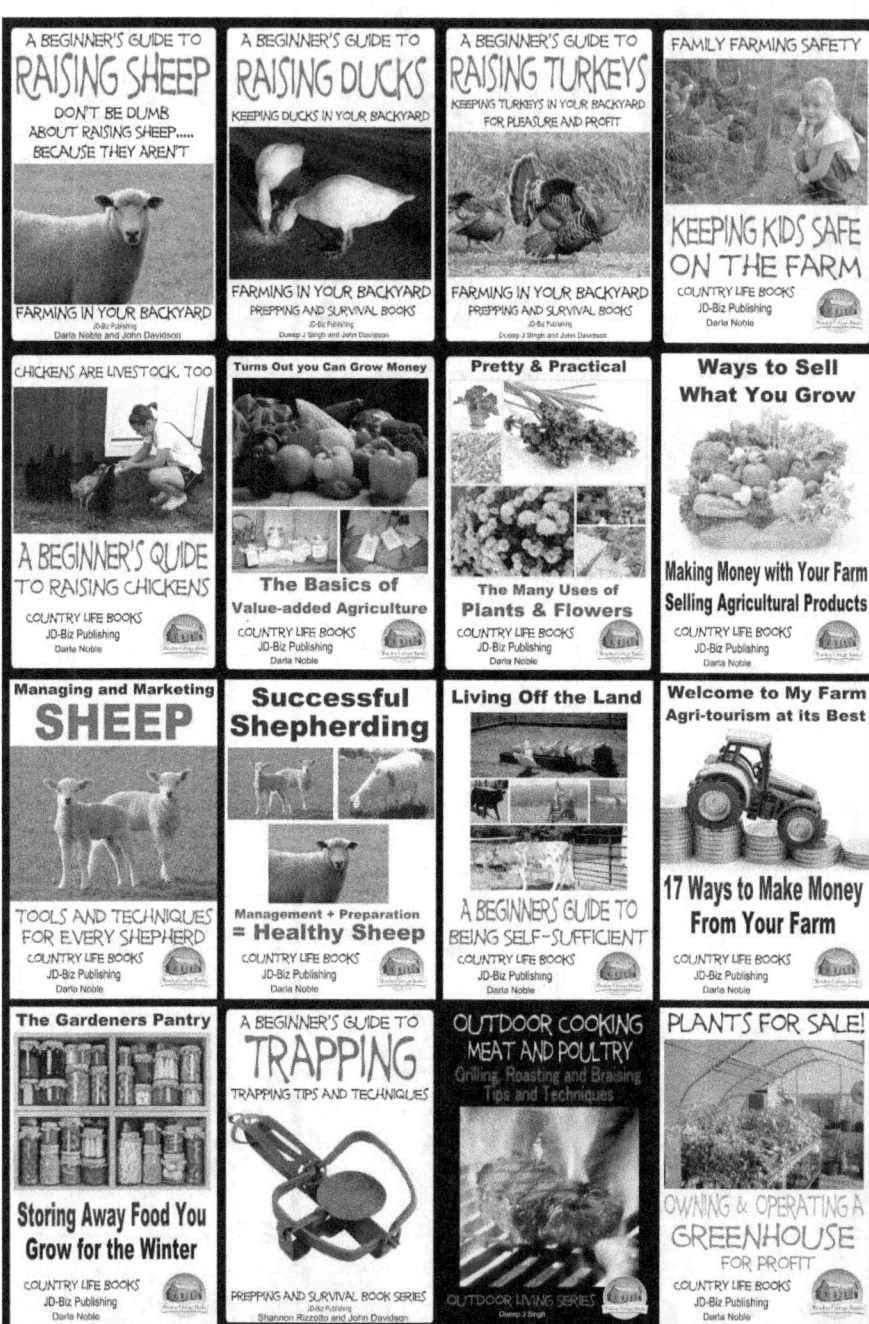

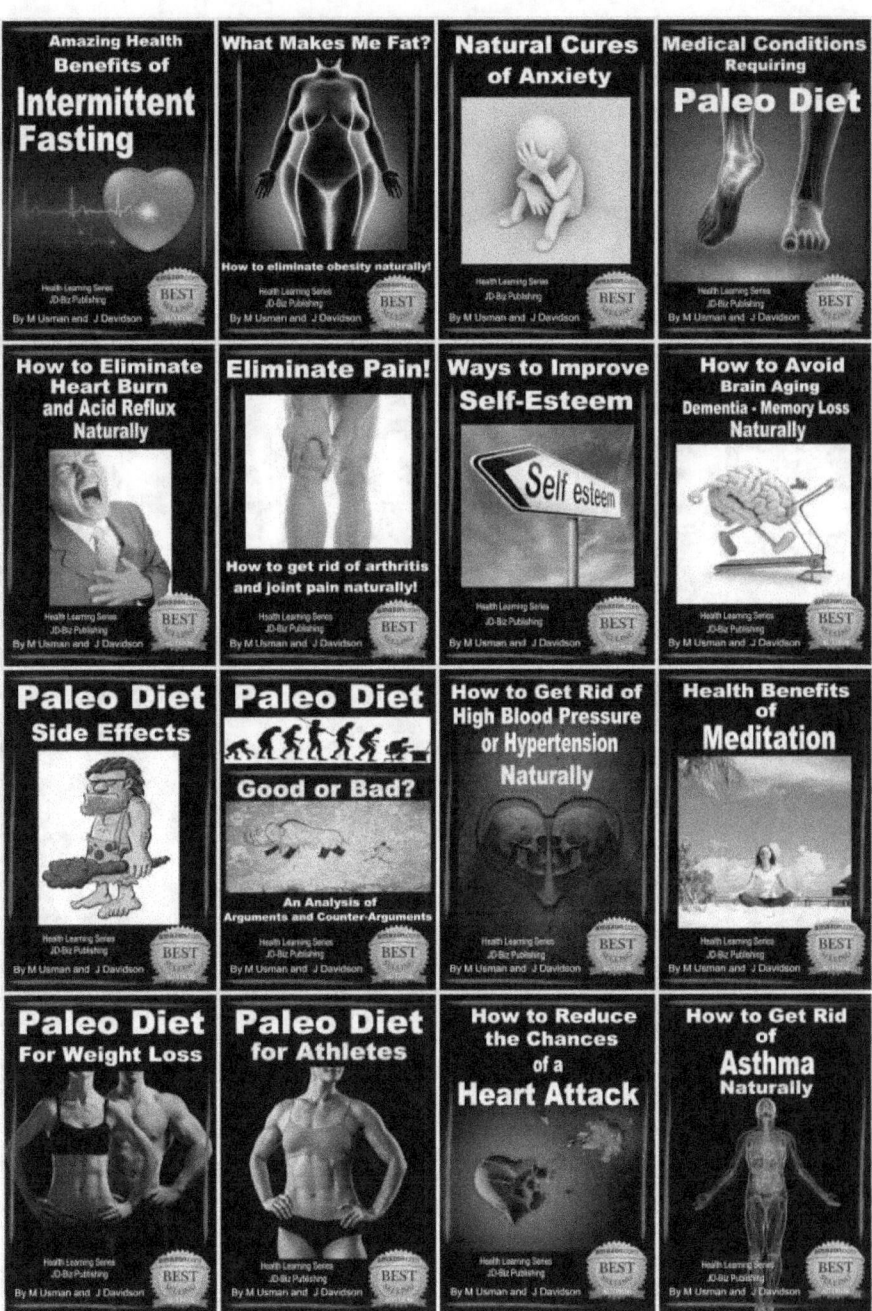

Chinchillas · Beavers · Snakes · Dolphins · Wolves · Walruses
Polar Bears · Turtles · Bees · Frogs · Horses · Monkeys
Dinosaurs · Sharks · Whales · Spiders · Big Cats · Big Mammals of Yellowstone
Animals of Australia · Sasquatch - Yeti Abominable Snowman Bigfoot · Giant Panda Bears · Kittens · Komodo Dragons · Lady Bugs
Animals of North America · Meerkats · Birds of North America · Penguins · Hamsters · Elephants

Learn To Draw Series

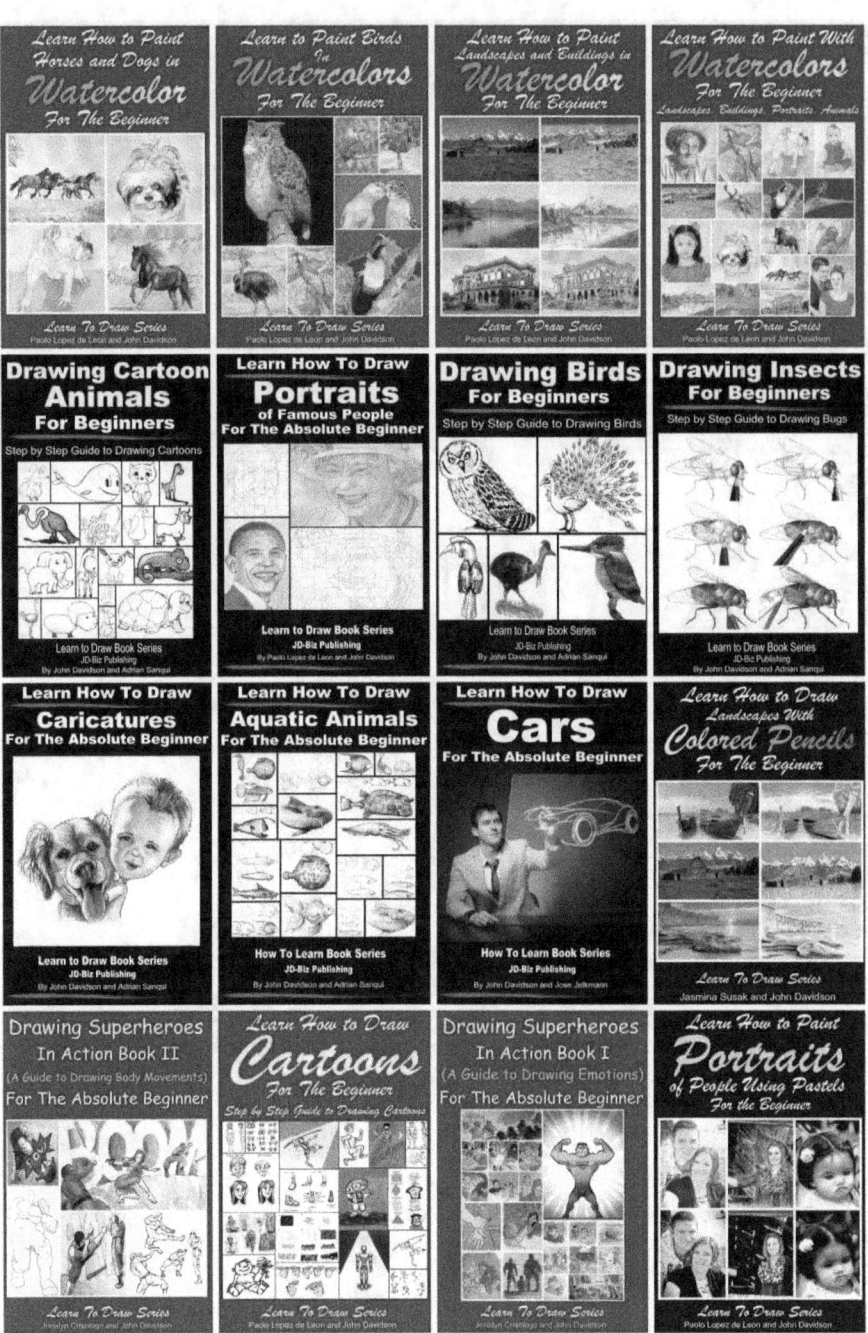

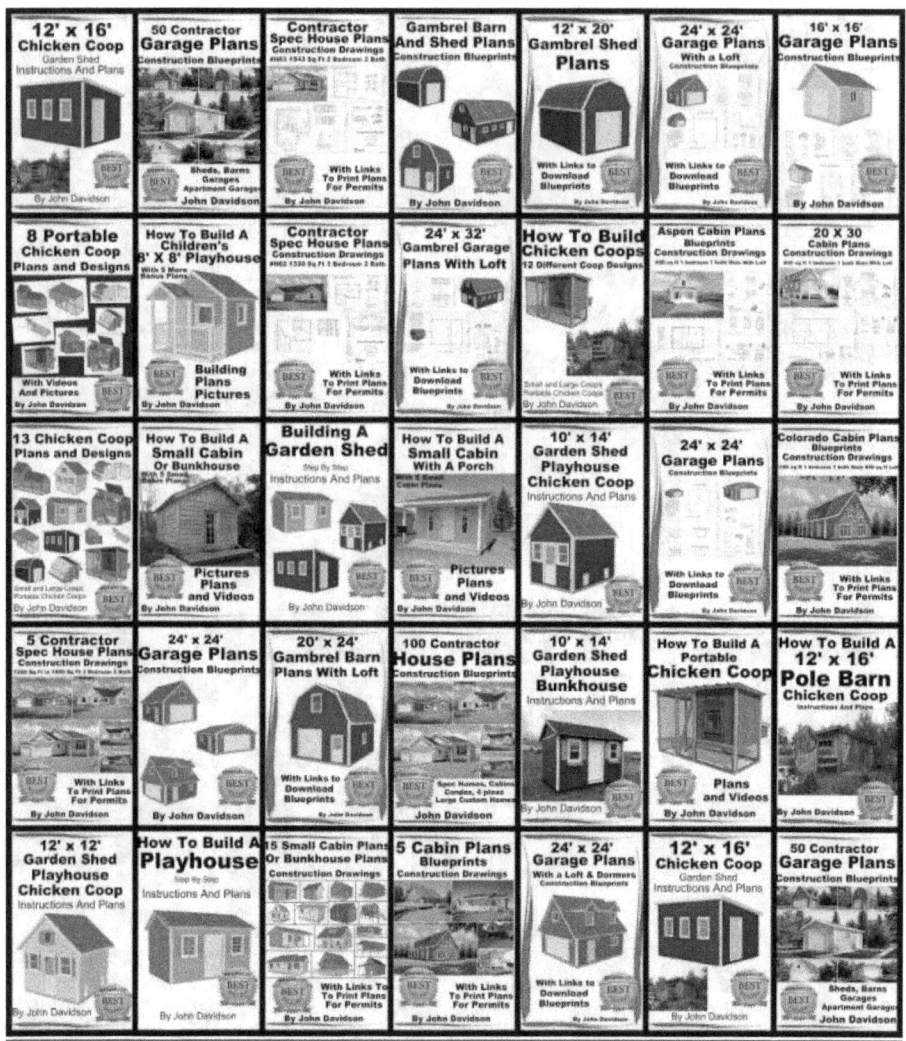

Entrepreneur Book Series

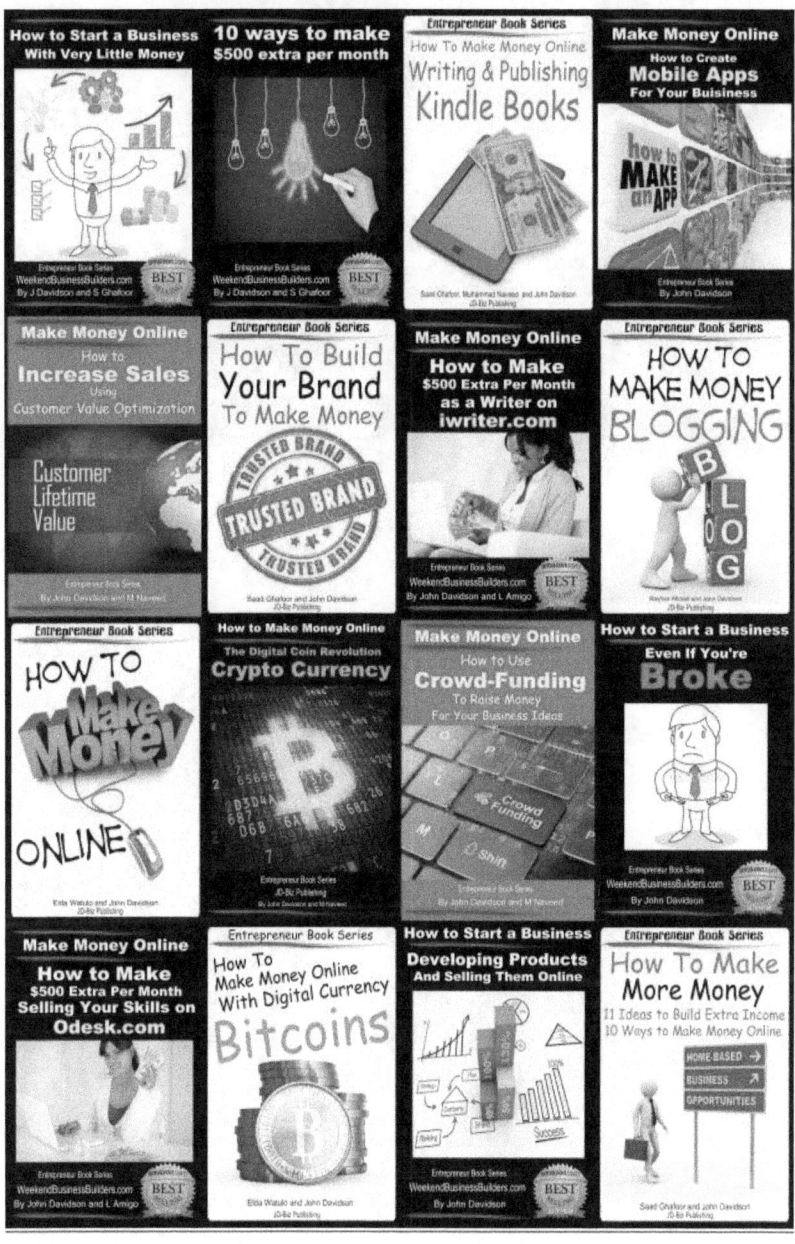

Our books are available at

1. Amazon.com

2. Barnes and Noble

3. Itunes

4. Kobo

5. Smashwords

6. Google Play Books

Publisher

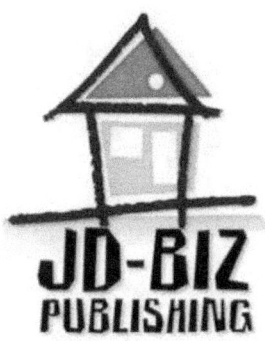

JD-Biz Corp

P O Box 374

Mendon, Utah 84325

http://www.jd-biz.com/

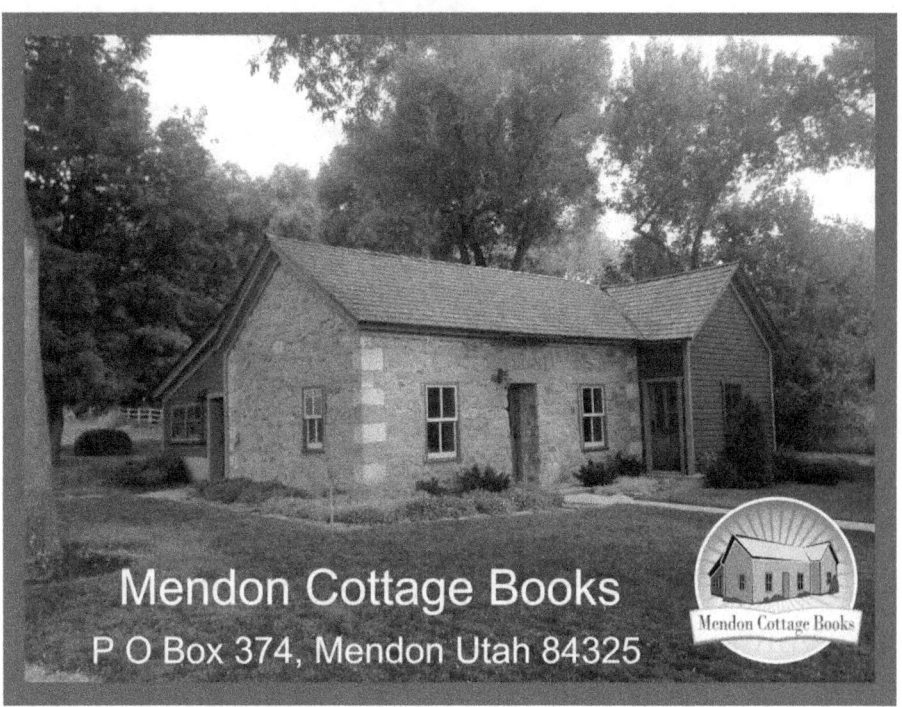

Mendon Cottage Books

P O Box 374, Mendon Utah 84325

Mendon Cottage Books

www.ingramcontent.com/pod-product-compliance
Lightning Source LLC
Chambersburg PA
CBHW070344290526
45791CB00003B/1465